How You Can Easily Make Hand Sanitizer at Home When All the Stores Run Short of It

Gladys Emo

Contents

INTRODUCTION

There is a recent spread of a deadly disease called COVID-19 which started in China, early in the year 2020. This COVID-19 otherwise called CORONA VIRUS spreads easily and quickly through human contact, and one of the best ways to control its spread is by constant washing of your hands. Hand sanitizer is seen to be also effective at eliminating bacteria and viruses, and you can carry a hand sanitizer anywhere you go, and you can use it when you are out and busy and nowhere close to a sink. This guide is to help you through how you can make your own hand sanitizer at home.

CHAPTER ONE: What you need to know

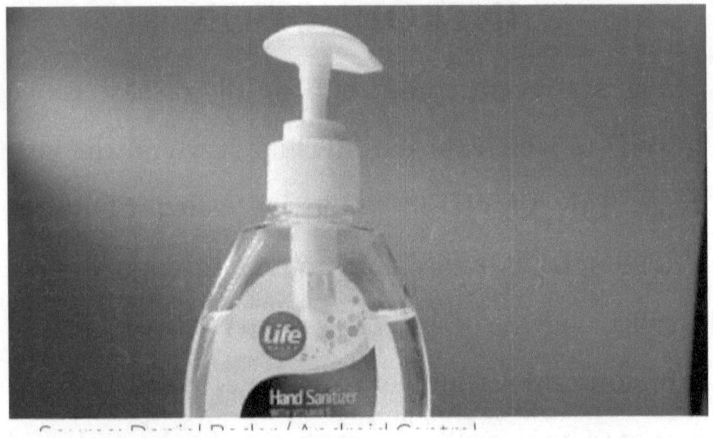

- A hand sanitizer is the only option you have in eliminating viruses when you are out of your house, or out and busy and you can't possibly get access to a sink to wash your hands.

- The Center for Disease Control and Prevention (CDC) has recommended that the best way to protect yourself from the virus is to wash your hands for about 20seconds when you return from a public place.

- The general rule is that you should not touch your nose, your eyes or mouth with your hands when they are not washed.

- If you are using a hand sanitizer, that hand sanitizer must contain at least 60% (sixty percent) of alcohol. The reason for this recommendation is because some hand sanitizers do not contain alcohol at all.

- Hand sanitizers without alcohol can never be effective in eliminating bacteria and viruses like the one that has enough alcohol.

- The appropriate way to use a hand sanitizer is to apply it generously to your hands and rub them together until the gel becomes even on your skin.

- The demand for hand sanitizers has increased greatly within a short period of time, because of the deadly Corona virus epidemic. So, in case you are running short of some, here is how you can easily make some at home.

List of Ingredients required in making hand sanitizer

A hand sanitizer requires just a simple formula and it consists of only few ingredients. It is also very easy to make your own at home if the pharmacy around you is running out of same. These are the ingredients you will need.

(1)   **2/3 cup 99.9% Isopropyl alcohol or 190-proof grain alcohol**

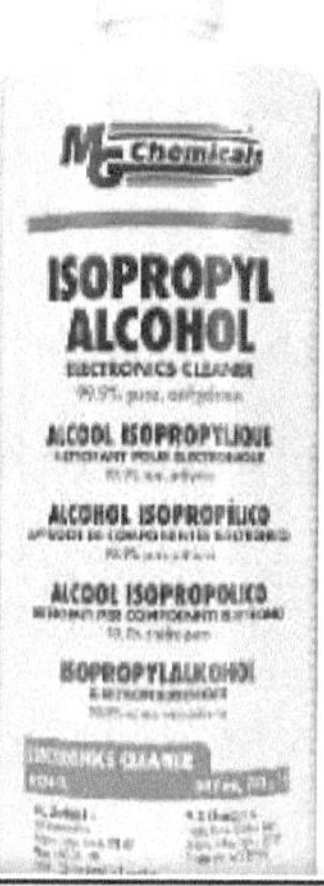

You can find Isopropyl alcohol at any local drug store or pharmacy. Your sanitizer mix must have at least 60% of alcohol for it to be effective. But I will advise that you get one that has more than 60%. A bottle of 99% alcohol is preferable and perfect for the mix. A one-quarter bottle can be purchased for around $15, and with that, you can make a lot of hand sanitizer. To be on the safer side, you can decide to buy a six-quarter pack.

(2)   1/3 cup 98% pure aloe vera gel (preferably without additives)

Isopropyl must be mixed with something. The reason is because on its own it's very harsh on the skin and it will burn your hands. So, the appropriate solution is to use aloe vera gel to mix the isopropyl, as aloe vera gel is a natural moisturizer.

(3)   8-10 drops of essential oils

In case you feel like adding some fragrance to the mixture, just buy a pack of essential oils. It could either be clove, cinnamon, lavender or peppermint. Although this is not needed, but most of the packet hand sanitizers sold these days have some fragrance. And if you are used to the smell, then there is no harm in picking up a few essential oils.

(4) Bowl and Spoon to mix it all together

(5) A basic funnel to pour the hand sanitizer into a bottle

(6) Plastic travel bottles- for storing the sanitizer.

When your hand sanitizer is ready, you will need bottles/containers to store it in. you can buy a six pack of 2oz bottles for like $7 (dollars) and they usually come with a flip top that makes it easy to squeeze out the hand sanitizer. Six pack of 8oz bottles can be bought for $9 (dollars).

(7) Nitrile Gloves

You need the nitrile gloves, so that you don't burn your hands when making the sanitizer. The Isopropyl alcohol is highly inflammable and it will burn your skin, if it happens to come into direct contact with your hands, so using nitrile gloves is highly recommended as a general precaution.

Once you are ready to start, ensure your tools for mixing are properly sanitized, or else you could contaminate the whole thing. Also, the WHO has recommended that you let your mixture stay for a minimum of 72 hours after you are done. That way, the sanitizer will have time to eliminate any bacteria that might have entered during the mixing process. Now, here is what you need to do:

Instructions

1.   Prepare the hand sanitizer in a very clean space. Wipe down the counter tops with a diluted bleach solution beforehand.

2.   Make sure you wash your hands thoroughly before making the hand sanitizer.

3.   To mix, make sure you use a clean spoon to whisk. And ensure you wash these items thoroughly before you start using them.

4.   Check well to be sure the alcohol used for the hand sanitizer is not diluted.

5.   When you mix all the ingredients together, do it thoroughly until they are well blended.

6.   And make sure you don't touch the mixture with your hands until it is ready for use.

Take Note: Hand sanitizers can be made in different formulas, whichever you prefer. You can choose either alcohol or witch-hazel & tea-tree-oil sanitizer. Let us take a look at how to make these two formulas below

Alcohol-Based Hand Sanitizer

Put your ingredients together

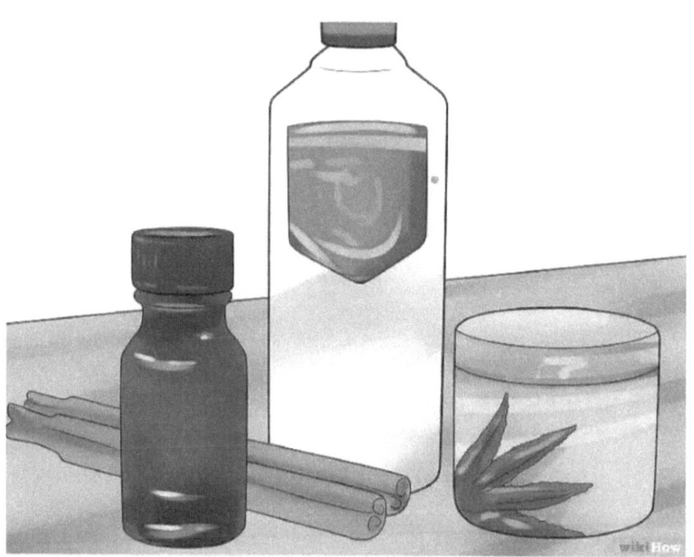

Directions

1.   **Pour the isopropyl alcohol and aloe vera gel into a bowl and use spoon to mix them.**

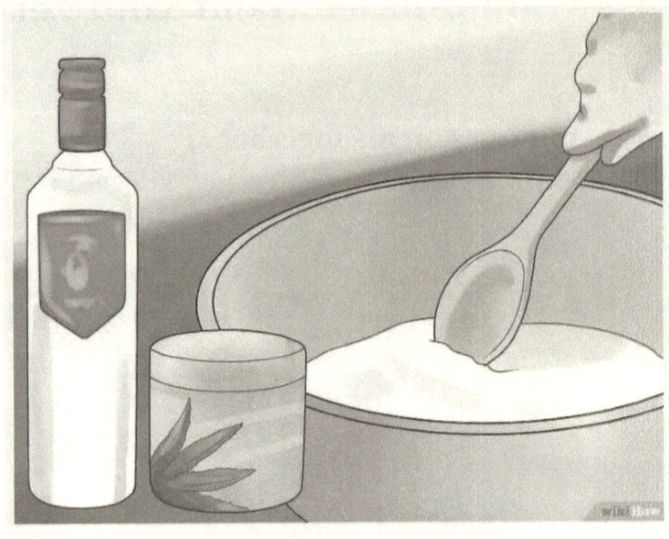

•   Make the mixture to be completely smooth.

•   If you want a thicker solution, add an extra spoonful of aloe vera.

•   But if you want your mixture to be lighter, add another spoonful of alcohol.

Since hand sanitizers need at least 60% of alcohol for it to be effective, then ideally, you should maintain an isopropyl alcohol to aloe vera gel ratio of 2:1. So, if you add 2oz of isopropyl alcohol, you should mix it with 2oz of aloe vera gel.

2.   **Add essential oils to the mix if needed.** You don't really need essential oils, but if you like a particular smell, you can add little drops of oil.

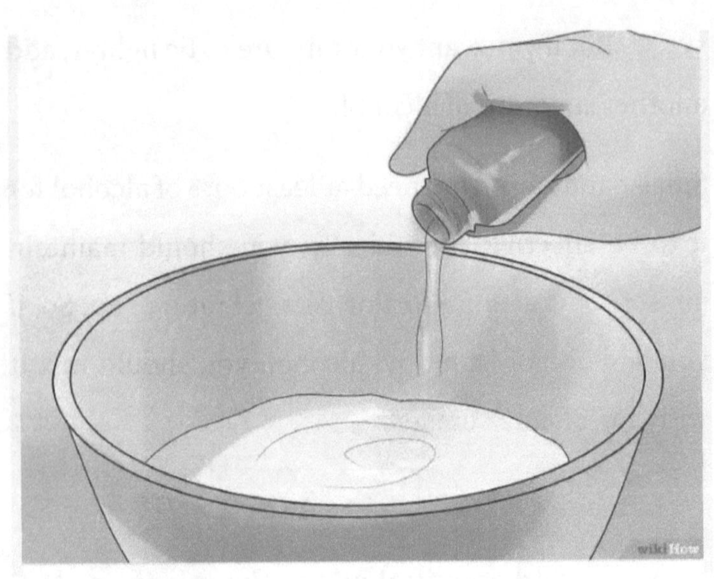

•   The right procedure is to add one drop at a time, and be stirring it as you add.

•   After adding like 8 drops, smell the mixture to know whether you like the scent. If the smell is strong enough, stop adding.

•   If you want the scent to be stronger, add some more drops.

•   Essential oils like Lavender, clove, cinnamon and peppermint have extra benefit of providing additional antiseptic properties to the mixture.

•   If you don't like any of these scents, you are free to use whatever scent you prefer. You can either choose Lemon, grapefruit or passion fruit, they all smell good.

3.   **Stir the ingredients together with a spoon and pour them into plastic bottles using a funnel.**

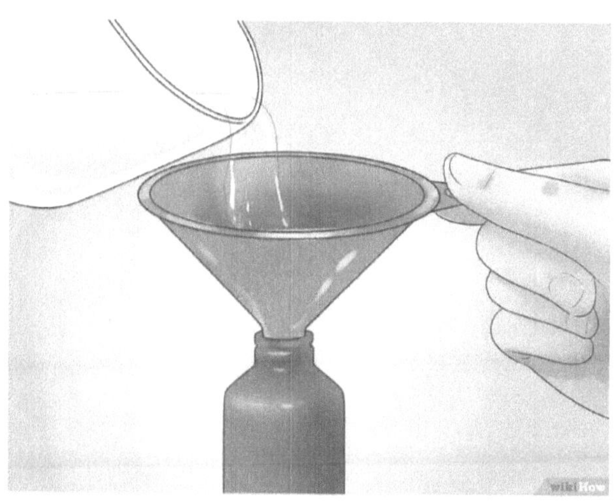

Put the funnel on top the mouth of the container, and pour the hand sanitizer into it. Fill the container up, and then tighten the lid until you are ready to use it.

•	You can use a small squirt bottle. It is actually handy, if you want to carry the sanitizer with you throughout the day.

•	If the hand sanitizer you made is too much for the bottle, you can save the leftover in a jar that has a tightly-fitted lid.

Your hand sanitizer is now ready for your use.

CHAPTER TWO: Witch Hazel-Based Hand Sanitizer

1.   Put your ingredients together.

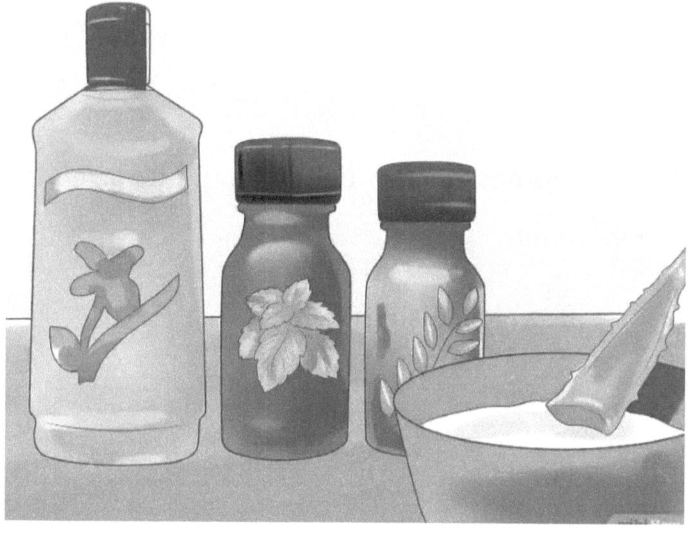

Due to the fact that alcohol has a strong smell and can severely dry the skin, some people prefer not to use alcohol when making their hand sanitizer. So an alternative such persons have is to make a witch-hazel based sanitizer. Tea tree oil is what you will use to make the witch-hazel based sanitizer and this tea tree oil provides additional antiseptic benefits to it. Below is a list of what you will need.

•   1 cup of pure aloe vera gel it's best without additives).

•   1 ½ tea spoons witch hazel 30 drops of tea tree oil

•   5 drops of essential oil, could be lavender or peppermint

•   Bowl for mixing

•   Spoon

•   Funnel

•   Plastic container

2.   **Mix the aloe vera gel, tea tree oil and witch hazel by stirring with a spoon**

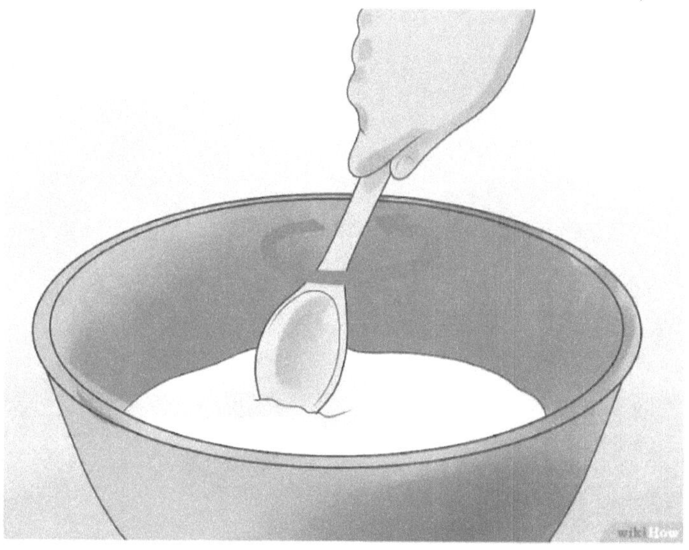

If the mixture is too thin, add an extra spoonful of aloe vera to make it thick. And if it is too thick, add an extra spoonful of witch hazel.

3. **Turn in the essential oil and Stir**

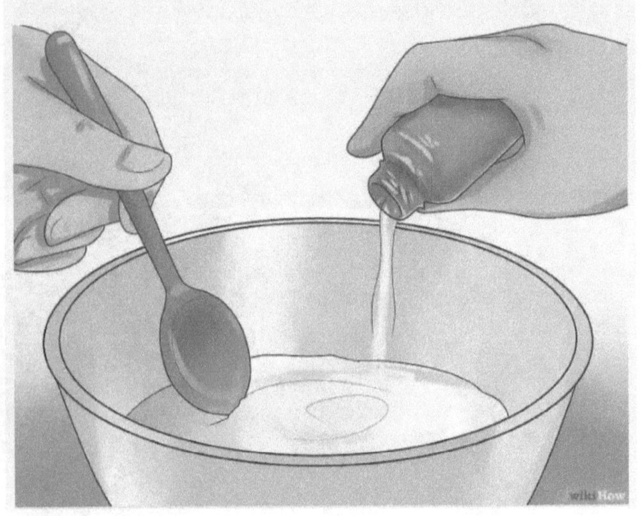

Tea tree oil is usually very strong, so make sure the essential oils you add is not too much. Like five drops should be enough, but if you want to add more, then add one drop at a time, stir it as you do so.

4.   **Turn the mixture into the container by using a funnel**

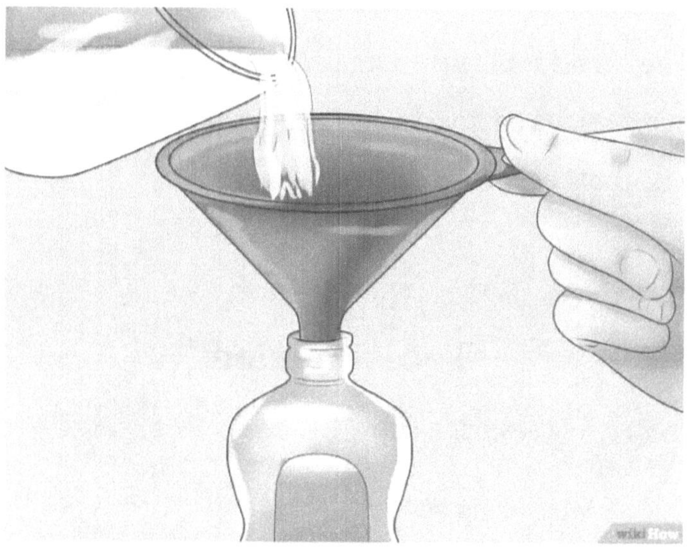

Put the funnel on the mouth of the container and pour the hand sanitizer in. make sure you fill it up, then close and tighten the lid until you are ready to use it.

- You can use a small squirt bottle, especially if you want to carry the sanitizer about with you when you are out and busy.

- If the sanitizer you made is too much and cannot all be contained in the bottle, save the leftover sanitizer in a jar that has a tightly-fitted lid.

The World Health Organization has also given instructions on how to make Hand Sanitizer at home. The tools needed are listed below

Tools Needed

- A Measuring cup

- Measuring spoons

- Whisk

- Spray bottles (empty ones)

- Sanitizer containers (empty ones) (needed for gel formulation)

INGREDIENTS

- 1 cup of 99% isopropyl alcohol

- 1 tablespoon of 3% hydrogen peroxide

- 1 teaspoon of 98% glycerin

- 85 milliliters of sterile boiled water.

The World Health Organization (W.H.O) has an extensive guide on how to make your own hand sanitizer. The only disadvantage with this formula is that if you follow this instruction, you will end up having a lot of it. You may end up with exactly 2.6 gallons of it. If you want to make enough hand sanitizer to last for you, your family and all your friends, you definitely can. But if you want to make a smaller quantity, I have adapted the measurements for you.

DIRECTIONS

1.   **Turn the alcohol into a container of medium size using a pouring spout.**

The percentages that is on the labels of isopropyl alcohol, states the level of alcohol concentration in them. Take note that you are dealing with almost pure alcohol if you have got 99.8%, but if it is 70% alcohol it means the bottle is only a little more than two-thirds (2/3) alcohol, and the rest is just water.

Some people have tried to adopt for their formulations the proportion of using 91% isopropyl alcohol or even 70%. But take note that these alcohol concentrations will render a final product that doesn't comply with the CDC's recommendation of using hand sanitizer with at least 60% alcohol to fight the COVID-19 ineffective.

2.   **Add hydrogen peroxide**

Hydrogen peroxide is a type of antiseptic and it is used on the skin for prevention against infection of minor wounds, scrapes and burns. It works by releasing oxygen when it is applied to an affected area, in this case it will be added to the mix. And when added, the release of oxygen will cause the mixture to foam. The hydrogen peroxide in the mixture is very effective in removing dead skin.

3.   **Add the glycerin and stir.**

Glycerin is thicker than both alcohol and hydrogen peroxide, so you will have to stir for some time to be able to combine everything together. You need a clean spoon to do this or, if your container has a lid, you can put that on, make sure you shake it very well.

4.   **Measure and pour in the water**

If you want to use 99% of isopropyl alcohol, you have to measure ¼ of a cup, 1 tablespoon of distilled or boiled cold water and add it all to your mixture. But if you are using an isopropyl alcohol that is less than 99%, you should pour enough water so as to get to a final volume of 345 milliliters, or approximately 1.4 cups. Then stir your mixture.

5.   Your spray bottles must be sanitized before you pour in your hand sanitizer.

Pour some of your leftover alcohol into your bottles and let them stay until the alcohol has evaporated. Then pour in your sanitizer.

6.   Label your bottles.

To avoid accidents, like a case where you or anybody else ingests the newly made hand sanitizer, the take the time to label your bottles appropriately. When your bottles are properly labeled, your chances of mistaking one of these for a flask will be slim, but of course accidents do happen.

CHAPTER THREE: How to Use Your Hand Sanitizer

There are two important things to take note of when using your hand sanitizer. The first thing is that you need to rub it into your skin until your hands are dry. Secondly, if your hands are greasy or dirty, you must first wash them with soap and water before you apply your hand sanitizer.

Having that in mind, here are some few tips on how to use hand sanitizer effectively.

1.   You can either spray or apply the sanitizer to the palm of your hand.

2.   Rub your hands together thoroughly. Ensure the sanitizer covers the entire surface of your hands and all your fingers.

3.   Rub continuously for like 30 to 60 seconds or until your hands are dry. It can take up to 60seconds

or more and sometimes longer for hand sanitizer to kill most germs

What Germs Can Hand Sanitizer Kill

Based on CDC's research, an alcohol-based hand sanitizer which meets the alcohol requirement can easily reduce the number of microbes and bacteria on your hands. It can also help to eliminate a wide range of disease-causing agents or pathogens on your hands, including the now common corona virus (COVID-19).

Important Things to Note

Keep in mind that even the best hand sanitizer that is alcohol-based have limitations and do not eliminate all types of germs.

According to the CDC, hand sanitizers will not get rid of chemicals that are potentially harmful. It is also not effective at killing the germs listed below:

- Clostridium difficile (also known as C.diff)

- Norovirus

- Cryptosporidium (which causes cryptosporidiosis)

Also take note that a hand sanitizer may not be effective if your hands are visibly dirty or greasy. This could be as a result of after eating food, doing yard work, gardening or playing a sport.

If your hands are or look dirty or slimy, go for hand washing instead of a hand sanitizer.

Hand washing vs. Hand sanitizer

It is important and helpful to know when is best to wash your hands, and when a hand sanitizer can be helpful. This is the key you need to note in protecting yourself from the novel corona virus as well as other illnesses, such as the common cold and seasonal flu.

Although both systems serve a purpose, but washing your hands with soap and water must always be a priority, this is based on the CDC recommendation. You should only use hand sanitizer if your soap and water isn't available in a particular situation.

You should wash your hands after doing any of the under listed:

- After going to the bathroom

- After blowing your nose, coughing or sneezing

- Before eating

☐   After touching surfaces that could be contaminated.

The CDC has given specific instructions on the best and most effective way to wash your hands. This is their recommendation:

1.   Ensure you use clean, running water always. (it can be warm or cold)

2.   First wet your hands, then turn the water off and rub soap on your hands

3.   Rub the soap on your hands together for at least 20 seconds. Ensure you scrub the back of your hands, between your fingers an under your nails.

4.   Turn on the water and rinse your hands. Then use a clean towel or air dry.

Frequently Asked Questions (Faq)

(1)   How long does it take to prepare a hand sanitizer?

It takes only about fifteen (15) to twenty (20) minutes to prepare.

(2)   Can the Hand Sanitizer be used in a Hospital site in a developing country?

Yes, it is acceptable to use a hand sanitizer in a hospital site in a developing country, if you don't have anything better to use.

(3)   Can I make the hand sanitizer slimy?

Just spread out the hand sanitizer you made on to a plate, then place it in the freezer, for like two to three hours. It will become slimy after a while.

(4)   Between the Alcohol and Witch-Hazel, which is better for Hand Sanitizer?

It is preferable to make an alcohol-based hand sanitizer, as alcohol is very effective in killing germs, bacteria and viruses, as previously discussed.

(5)   Can I prepare my Hand sanitizer without Aloe Vera and Peppermint?

Yes, you can prepare your hand sanitizer without any of the two. Water can be used as the base and then, you can use any essential oil of your choice other than peppermint if you don't like the smell, or you could also decide not to use any oil at all.

(6)   How long can a home-made hand sanitizer last in a jar?

If you keep it in the appropriate temperature, it will last for a couple of months, the alcohol in it will act as a preservative.

(7)   Is it possible that the essential oils will cover the smell of the alcohol?

Definitely, the smell of the essential oils you add to your sanitizer will outshine the smell of the alcohol.

(8)   Where can I find these ingredients to make the hand sanitizer?

You can get the ingredients from any local pharmacy, also some department stores too could possibly have. You can also get them from a grocery store but take note that it may be more expensive there.

(9)   For someone who is allergic to aloe vera, what can he/she possibly use?

Vegetable Glycerine can be used as a substitute to Aloe Vera

(10)   Can 70% alcohol be used, if 99% alcohol is not available?

You can use 70% alcohol, but make sure you don't add anything to it. Then leave it on the skin to dry. Thereafter, add normal hand cream to it.

CONCLUSION

It is handy to go with a hand sanitizer, to help you prevent the spread of germs in a situation where soap and water is not available. Hand sanitizers that are alcohol based can help keep you safe and reduce the spread of the new disease called corona virus.

So, if you can't find hand sanitizers at your local stores, you can take these steps explained above to make your own. All you need are few ingredients, such as rubbing alcohol, aloe vera gel and an essential oil or lemon juice.

Though hand sanitizers can be effective in getting rid of germs, however Health Authorities still recommend "hand washing" as much as possible to keep your hands free of viruses that causes diseases and other germs.

So, washing your hands with soap and water is the best option, but if you have no soap and water, hand sanitizer is the second-best option. Hand sanitizers sold commercially, can become expensive, and with the shortage of hand sanitizer due to recent outbreak of COVID-19, your only option may just be to make your own in your home.